THE POWER OF PLANTS

HOW FOOD AND CANNABIS HELPED ME HEAL

BAINTI PARMAR

I want to dedicate this book to my mom, whose sacrifices made my journey to health possible. Thank you for enduring countless sleepless nights, for shedding so many tears of worry. You lived each pain with me, and you were even happier than I was when I could walk again. Your tireless efforts are the reason I'm writing this book. Your strength and faith kept me going. I love you so very much.

ONE

At least you have your health—that's what people often say to console you when you hit a rough patch in your life. *I'm sorry you lost your job, but at least you have your health. Too bad about the bankruptcy, but at least you have your health.* No one ever said that to me though, not that I can remember, because I never really had my health. As a child, I was constantly getting sick or hurt, so much so that I was known as the "unwell one," and that was before I was diagnosed with type 1 diabetes when I was nine years old, living in Delhi, India.

In the months before my diagnosis, I remember being tired all the time. My older sister and my younger brother ran around all day, playing with each other inside our house or with our friends out in the neighborhood, but I just couldn't find the energy to keep up with them. It hadn't always been that way. Before I turned nine, we ran around together for hours and hours every day. My sister and I were constantly playing games and sports. But after my ninth birthday, I struggled to get off the couch. I felt like a toy robot whose batteries were slowly dying. Every movement had become a struggle for me.

My parents thought my low energy and the weight I'd gained in the preceding months were due to my laziness. Whenever I told them that I didn't want to go outside to play, they scolded me, telling me to quit making excuses and to get out there and get some exercise. They are very loving people, and I know they thought they were doing what was best for me, but it bothered me when they told me to stop being lazy. I really wanted to play outside, but my body seemed to have developed a mind of its own. I just couldn't budge it.

On the day of my diagnosis, I remember feeling especially tired on my way to school. My energy levels were so low that even sitting at my desk was a challenge. And when it was time for PE class, I shuffled outside to play in our schoolyard. I wanted to do anything but play, but school rules were school rules, so I trudged through our exercises. I was relieved when we went back to class.

While I was sitting at my desk after PE, I started to feel weak and dizzy. I told my teacher that I didn't feel well, and she sent me to the nurse's office. The nurse gave me some glucose and instructed me to lie down for a while. I did as I was told, and for the next half hour, I lay on a cot, staring up at the ceiling, wondering what my friends were doing in class.

Thirty minutes later, the nurse asked me to sit up. I told her that I still didn't feel well, but she said that I'd be fine, and she sent back to class.

I sat at my desk for a few minutes, trying my best to pay attention to what the teacher was saying, but I couldn't focus. I asked her if I could go back to the nurse's office. I must have looked pretty ill because she didn't question me. She told me that I could lie down for as long as I needed to.

On my way back to the nurse's office, I blacked out. I was walking down the hallway one minute, and the next minute I was waking up on the cot in the nurse's office. It was clear to the nurse now that I was actually not well, and she called my mom to pick me up.

I was absent from school for the next two days so my mom could take me to see a doctor. I had blood drawn for tests that would determine what was wrong with me. I hated the poking and prodding, but I could tell from the look on my mom's face that she was really concerned. I didn't want her to worry more than she already was, so I sat still while the lab tech sucked out my blood like a giant mosquito.

A couple days after our visit to the doctor's office—July 15, 2002, to be exact—our family doctor called my house around 7:00 in the evening and asked my mom to take me to his office immediately. My mom was a bit freaked out, and I know she would have appreciated support from my dad, but he was on a business trip in Germany at the time. I could tell from her reaction to the doctor's call that the news wasn't good, but I remember being more concerned for her than I was for myself. I hated seeing her so upset.

We left my siblings with a family member, then we headed to our doctor's office. Inside the exam room, the doctor sat us both down and told my mom that I had type 1 diabetes. I had no idea what diabetes was, but my mom had tears in her eyes, so I assumed that it was something serious. The doctor told her that my sugar level was over 600 mg/dL, which was significantly higher than the target range of 100-180 mg/dL for that age at that time of day. The doctor told my mom that he was seriously concerned for my health, and he recommended that I immediately go to the hospital so I could be admitted. We left minutes later, heading home first to pack a bag for a stay in the hospital. My mom cried the whole way.

I was admitted that night. My mom must have thought that I was at death's doorstep because every time I woke up in the middle of the night, she was looking down on me, wide awake. That must have been a horrifying night for her, especially since my dad wasn't there to share her pain.

I stayed in that hospital for a full week. The tedium of sitting all day was interrupted occasionally by visits from worried family members, whose faces all looked as distraught as my mother's. My dad cut his work in Germany short and hurried back to Delhi to be at my bedside. I was happy to see him when he arrived, but I hated to see the tears in his eyes. Everyone around me was crying, which was a little confusing because I was starting to feel better. The medicine that the nurses gave me was obviously doing the trick, and I had more energy than I'd had in months.

One of the doctors in the hospital came by my room toward the end of my stay to give me a quick "diabetes education." He explained the causes of the disease, the dietary restrictions, the insulin injections. I was too young to understand everything he was saying, but it started to dawn on me why the people around me were so sad. I'd thought that I was going to be healed after I left the hospital, but the doctor was telling me that I had a disease that I was going to carry with me for the rest of my life. It was like he'd handed me a backpack full of bricks and told me that I had to lug it around everywhere I went, forever. I know it's irrational, but I resented that doctor. His news completely changed the way I looked at the world and at my place in it. I had a disease. My body was flawed. And if I didn't follow the regimen they laid out for me, I could get seriously sick or die. It wasn't fair.

My new life started the day I left the hospital. Besides all the rules about what I could and couldn't eat, I also had to have insulin injections every day, four times a day. Four times a day! I had to sit there and let my mom jab me with a needle more times every day than most people brush their teeth. And my mom had to check my blood sugar levels three to five times a day by pricking my finger with a lancet, a small, sharp needle that was designed specifically to make fingers bleed. It was like a torture device meant to make the lives of children miserable.

Another downside of the disease was that everyone and their mother dropped by our home to give me advice about how to cure or cope with diabetes. It was as if my diagnosis had coincided with the graduation of dozens of new doctors in my neighborhood. Everyone was suddenly an expert. Eat this; don't eat that. Definitely don't drink that. The people who visited to share their unsolicited advice meant well, but they really had no idea what they were talking about. They didn't know much about type 1 diabetes because the disease wasn't as common then as it is now. The sad fact is that there are an estimated 420 million type 1 diabetics in the world today, and that number is rising. The disease has become all too familiar to far too many people since I was diagnosed sixteen years ago, and it looks like there are going to be a lot more little girls like me whose lives are going to change drastically with their diagnoses.

Not long after arriving back home after my stay in the hospital, I started to resent all the tears people shed over me when they came for a visit. I was already feeling lousy about being told that I had a disease that would last forever. The pity of the people who visited just made me feel worse. I appreciated those guests who came by with a smile on their faces and who talked about anything but my diet and my injections. I remember wishing that my mom could somehow screen our guests so that only people without tears in their eyes would be allowed in to see me.

After the trauma of the diagnosis wore off, my parents decided that it was time to get me back to my studies, so we packed my bag and headed back to my school. Our first stop was the principal's office. My parents wanted to make him aware of my disease and to let him know that I might need extra attention from now on. The principal obviously knew nothing about diabetes, and he didn't seem interested in learning about it. He told my parents that sick children weren't allowed back at school and that they should keep me at home until I was well again. He seemed to think that diabetes was a communicable disease like TB or whooping cough. My parents eventually convinced him to allow me to continue coming to school in spite of my disease, but he wasn't willing to offer me any extra care. My mom had to stay in the school's waiting area while I was in class so she could help me with my injections. Needless to say, my parents weren't going to be nominating him for any principal of the year awards.

At home, my mom started doing some research into diets that were supposed to help me regulate my blood sugar level. She started introducing me to all sorts of alternative drinks: lemon juice, bitter gourd juice, Ayurvedic juices, Fenugreek juice. I didn't mind drinking some of those juices, but some of them tasted terrible. My mom encouraged me to pinch my nose and chug them down, promising that they would be good for me in the long run. I did as she asked, but I complained the whole time. Looking back on those days now, I wish I would have whined less to my mom. My disease was already hard enough on her without my moaning and groaning. But I suppose we all regret the way we sometimes acted toward our parents, even those of us who didn't have diseases.

I wish I could say that my mom discovered a miracle juice that helped me maintain my glucose level, but the truth is that nothing she asked me to drink did me any good. In the end, the only thing that helped were those painful insulin injections. I would have given anything to stop getting poked four times a day, but a reprieve wasn't in my cards.

About a year after my diagnosis, we learned about an insulin pump, a small pager-looking device that acts like a pancreas. You wear the pump around your waist, and it delivers insulin into your body through a catheter placed under the skin (ouch!). The downside of the pump is that you have to walk around all day every day with a catheter piercing the skin of your abdomen, held in place by a patch; the upside is that you don't have to get insulin injections four times a day (but with either delivery method, you still have to prick your fingers to check your glucose level). I liked the idea of avoiding those needles, and so did my parents. I don't think their distaste for giving me those shots could match my distaste for receiving them, but they clearly hated causing me pain, even if that pain was meant to keep me healthy. We all decided that we'd give the insulin pump a try at the earliest opportunity.

It turned out that the earliest opportunity was a couple years and half a world away.

TWO

My family and I moved to California—the East Bay, specifically—in 2004, when I was twelve. My parents thought we'd have a brighter future in the United States than in India, in part because I'd have access to better healthcare. It would be difficult for us to leave everything we'd ever known to live in a new country, but the pros of coming to the US far outweighed the cons.

I was both terrified and thrilled by the prospect of emigrating from India. I hated the thought of leaving so many friends and family members, but I did have two uncles living in the Bay Area, so we had some family support in the US. I was also excited to be moving to the state that gave us so many of the movies I loved to watch. And I couldn't wait to be around people who knew nothing of my medical history. I hated—hated!—that I was known as the "poor diabetic girl" in my community. The pity wore on my nerves. The thought of moving into a neighborhood where I was a complete unknown made my pulse quicken.

It was so surreal when we arrived at our new home in

California. I'd come to the US a few times before to visit my uncles and their families, but the sights, sounds, and smells always seemed strange to me. They were all completely different from what I'd experienced in India. The streets were so wide, and the cars were so fast. There weren't piles of trash on the street. Besides the occasional dog, it was rare to see an animal wandering around the city, and there were certainly no cows anywhere in sight. Everything seemed so tidy and manicured. It was definitely love at first sight, but I also instantly missed my life in Delhi. As beautiful as it was, this new country was going to take some getting used to.

My parents enrolled me in a middle school shortly after we arrived. The school was big and attractive, but I struggled to fit in initially. I was an incredibly shy girl, and I lacked the confidence necessary to walk up to someone and introduce myself. My shyness made it difficult for me to make new friends in my first few months of school.

But like many preteen dramas, the hard times didn't last forever for me. As the school year progressed, I started opening up to people, and I made several new friends, who all treated me kindly. I also came to know the school nurse fairly well. She knew much more about diabetes than the nurse in my school in India, and my mom didn't have to wait around to help me with my insulin shots. The nurse was more than capable of handling the shots by herself.

Not long after I started school, my parents got an insulin pump to help me regulate my blood sugar level. I was so ready to be done with those four daily shots, and it seemed that the pump would also afford me some more freedom and elbow room in my life. Like most twelve year olds, I was starting to get a little rebellious, and I wanted my parents to have less control over what I did and where I went.

My high school years were a much happier time for me in terms of my social life. I learned the art of making friends, and I was always surrounded by people who made me laugh and who shared memorable moments with me. Rallies, football and basketball games, dances, house parties—I took part in all the usual high school traditions that help students bond with their peers. When I look back on those years now, I feel blessed that I had so many wonderful people in my life. My friends made getting out of bed a joy most days.

I wish I could say that I was as careful about maintaining my health as I was about maintaining my friendships. I'm embarrassed to say that I wasn't very responsible in high school when it came to food. I ate what my mom wanted me to eat when I was home or when we went out for a meal, but when I was at school or at a friend's house, I ate all the forbidden foods. I was enjoying life, and I didn't want to put limits on my happiness. I didn't like saying no when a friend offered me some junk food at lunch, so I rarely did. I didn't check my blood sugar level as often as I should have. I figured I could eat whatever I wanted because I had an insulin pump that regulated my blood sugar level for me. My health just wasn't my top priority at that point in my life. My doctors had informed me of the consequences of abusing my body, but they made those consequences seem so distant. They told me what would happen to my body when I was forty or fifty. I was only a teenager then, and forty or fifty seemed unimaginably far away. I wish I could go back and talk some sense into the teenage version of myself because I paid the price for my immaturity, and so did my poor parents.

As a result of my bad behavior, I ended up in the ER at least three times for ketoacidosis, a complication of diabetes caused by high levels of blood acids called ketones. If there is too much glucose in your blood and not enough insulin, your body begins to break down fat to fuel itself, which produces a buildup of ketones. The condition makes you feel extremely thirsty, weak, tired, and sometimes confused. And if left untreated, ketoacidosis can cause death. I regret that my irresponsibility caused my parents so much worry. I thought I was proving to everyone how grownup I was by pretending that my disease was no big deal, but I was really showing the world that I couldn't be trusted to make good decisions about my health.

Recognizing that I needed to make a change in order to stay out of the ER, my mom tried everything she could think of motivate me. One of her most interesting suggestions was that I join a diabetes mentorship program, where older kids took younger kids under their wings and tried to help them avoid the mistakes they'd made. The older kids met with kids who'd recently been diagnosed with diabetes, and they told them what life with diabetes was like and how best to cope with the disease. The program sounded like a great idea in theory, and I love the concept now, but at the time I just wasn't in a position to offer anyone any advice. I was still bitter about having diabetes, and I really didn't understand the reality of the disease. My doctors had told me that diabetes was for life, but I couldn't fathom that forever really meant forever. A part of me believed that this was just a temporary inconvenience. I'd grow out of diabetes the same way I'd grown out of old clothes. I think part of the reason that I wouldn't accept the truth was because type 1 diabetes used to be called juvenile diabetes, and in a few years, I wasn't going to be an juvenile any more. In my mind, adults couldn't have juvenile diabetes, so as soon as I reach adulthood, I'd be in the clear.

I was clearly in denial about my disease. My experiences in the hospital had obviously taught me that there could unpleasant side effects if I made bad decisions, but I hadn't yet accepted that the really unpleasant stuff could happen to me if I didn't respect the disease. Heart disease, strokes, blindness, tooth decay, gum infections, amputated limbs—the list of horrors goes on and on. I know that at some point a doctor sat me down and revealed all the ugliness, but I guess I never really allowed myself to take it in. It all just seemed so distant. Those things didn't happen to young girls. They happened to old people. My youth was my shield.

For me, the combination of teenage hormones and diabetes made me intolerable. My parents are beautiful, loving people, but I'm a little surprised that they didn't strangle me when I was in high school. I certainly would have deserved it.

THREE

After I graduated from high school, I went to college in San Francisco. Much like leaving India, I was both terrified and thrilled when the day came for me to move out of my parents' house. My parents and I had argued often while I was in high school, mostly about my refusal to change my eating habits and to stay on top of my diabetes, but I still cried the day they dropped me off at campus. I missed them before they even left my dorm room.

Then they decided that it was time for them to move back to India. They had some family in the US, including me obviously, but most of their family members were back in Delhi. Their siblings, aunts, uncles, cousins, their parents —they had far more people there than they had here. They felt that they'd helped me settle into a nice life, and now it was time for them to reconnect with the people they'd left behind. I was very sad to see them go, but I also understood their decision and didn't hold it against them.

When classes started and I got busy with my studies—and with parties on the weekends—the sadness about their departure waned. I made several close friends not long after my first semester began. We hung out together all the time, sometimes in the library, other times at parties on weekends. We were young and free, and we made most of the same mistakes that college students make when they're living away from home for the first time.

Most of my mistakes still centered around my health. I was slightly more cautious about what I ate and drank, and I was better about regularly checking my blood sugar level, but I still wasn't as disciplined as I should have been. My lax attitude toward my health caught up to me one night while I was out with my friends. We went to dinner, then headed out to a campus party. A couple hours later, I started to feel weak and lightheaded, so I left my friends at the party and went back to my dorm to get some rest. I figured that if I got a good night's sleep, I'd feel better in the morning. That just goes to show how oblivious I was to the damage I was doing to my body.

I woke up the next morning feeling just as lousy. I checked my blood sugar level several times, and it fluctuated between high and low all that day. I stayed in bed, thinking that I just needed some extra rest, but by the time dinner rolled around, I was feeling even worse. It was clear that I wasn't going to get better on my own. My friend Ashley checked in on me that day to see how I was doing, so I asked her to take me to the hospital. She drove me to the nearest ER and stayed with me through the night. She was so good to me, and I'm lucky that she was in my life.

I was once again diagnosed with ketoacidosis. My A1C test results, which show the percentage of red blood cells in the body that have sugars attached to them, came back at 10.8%. That's a really dangerous level, and I was angry at myself for letting my health deteriorate to such an unmanageable level. I called my parents from the hospital and told them about my condition. They were both incredibly worried and extremely upset. They were tired of seeing me in the hospital, and it frustrated them to no end to know that my lack of self-control was entirely to blame for these trips to the ER. As I lay there in my hospital bed for the umpteenth time, my parents gave me an ultimatum: I either had to change my ways, or I had to leave college and come back to India to live with them. They wanted this to be my last visit to the ER, and they were willing to take drastic measures to make that happen.

I'm not sure if it was the pain that I heard in my parents' voices or the threat of having to move back in with them—or maybe a little of both—but I actually listened to them this time. I was having the time of my life in college, and I definitely didn't want to leave my friends, but I also didn't want to end up back in the ER. I was just as tired of hospitals as my parents were, and I hated feeling sick after going on a carbohydrate bender. So I started following my endocrinologist's advice and acted like I actually had diabetes. I juiced, ate salads and fish, and avoided junk food. I stuck with the basic diabetic diet: lots of proteins and fats and not many carbs. I also got into the habit of checking my blood sugar frequently, and I took insulin when I was supposed to take it. On top of all that, I started frequenting one of the gyms on campus. My efforts paid off. My A1C came down to 9.6%. Although I still had room for improvement, I started feeling much more energetic, much less sickly, which isn't to say that everything was perfect. I still had some bad days, but there were more good days than bad ones.

I know I shouldn't have been surprised by the positive results of a healthy lifestyle, but that period in my life was something of a revelation to me. I saw what my life could be like if I was willing to take my doctor's advice and make changes to my habits. I promised myself that I would stop behaving like a child. I was legally an adult, and it was time that I started acting like one.

A few months into my junior year, my friend invited me to her birthday party at a club. I met a boy there named Arjun. He seemed nice, and we started talking. It was clear right away that we were a good match for each other. Our personalities mixed well, and we definitely had chemistry. Soon enough we were dating, and my life would never be the same.

When we first started talking, I was worried that if Arjun found out about my diabetes, he might not be interested in continuing our relationship. If you Google diabetes and read about how it can ravage your body later in life, you'll find some scary stuff. But I decided that I had to be completely upfront with him about my health and about how poorly I'd been treating my body. I told him all about the bouts of illness and the stays in the hospital. I was ashamed that I'd caused myself and my parents so much suffering, but he was much more forgiving than I was. He didn't bat an eye when I opened up to him, which made me like him all the more. By telling him everything about my disease, I guess you could say that I was testing Arjun to find out how he would respond. I'm happy to say that he passed with flying colors.

The closer we became, the more active Arjun became in the management of my disease. He started off by doing a lot of research about diabetes, then he took a more hands-on role, including reminding me constantly to check my blood sugar level and to take my insulin when I needed it. He did everything that he possibly could to show me that I was special to him, and it made a huge difference in the way I approached my health. I didn't want to disappoint him by ending up in the hospital because of a self-inflicted illness, and I didn't want to spend time in the hospital that I could have been spending with him. He was a wonderful boyfriend in so many ways, and he deserves much of the credit for my transformation in the coming years. By walking shoulder to shoulder with me, he gave me the strength I needed to take control of my health, to put away all the bad habits that were taking years off my life. I owe Arjun so much.

FOUR

Three years after starting college in San Francisco, I decided that I'd had enough of school. I was only a year away from graduating, but I just wasn't into my studies any more, and I had no idea what I really wanted to do with my life. I talked with my parents, telling them that I was confused and lost and that I didn't know what to do next. I hated the idea of wasting their money on a degree in a field that I wasn't really interested in. I also hated the idea of walking away when I was so close to the finish line, but the thought of another year of college made me feel sick. On top of that, I wanted to get my health squared away. I was twenty-two at the time, and I felt that I needed to seriously take control of my diabetes. I figured that it would be easier to do that if I left college.

I decided that I wanted to spend some time in India with my family. My parents were very open to the idea, so I made arrangements to fly out there in June of 2014. I was excited to return after being gone for a decade, but I was also concerned about what would happen to my relationship with Arjun. We'd only been dating for a few months at that point, but our relationship had blossomed very quickly. He was an amazing boyfriend who was such a strong supporter in every aspect of my life, and I had a hard time telling him that I wanted to return to India for a while to visit my family and to determine what I wanted to do with my life. We loved each other, but I was afraid that the distance and the time away from our relationship might dim that love. But true to form, Arjun was completely supportive when I finally told him about my desire to go. He knew that I needed to spend quality time with my family, and he told me that he was confident that our relationship was strong enough to survive a period of separation. Other people managed long-distance relationships, and we could too.

My siblings decided that they wanted to come back to Delhi with me as well. I really enjoy spending time with them, and I was glad that we could all make new memories in India. When we landed in Delhi in the middle of the night, I was a bundle of conflicting emotions. I loved being in a place that was so familiar—the smells instantly took me back to my childhood—but I also felt an emotional distance from the city, from the country really. I'd been in the US since I was twelve, which meant that I'd lived in the States for nearly as long as I'd lived in India. Returning to India didn't really feel like a homecoming because it wasn't my home any more. The city felt like an old friend I'd lost contact with over the years. I was happy that we were finally reunited, but there was a part of me that was sad to know I'd never have the kind of friendship we'd had in the past.

My family was a different story though. It was just straight bliss seeing my parents. It had been a couple years since they'd moved, and it was so nice to hug them again. I loved being with them all in the same place. It made me nostalgic for my youth.

While I was there, I was pretty disciplined when it came to food. I cheated every once in a while, but for the most part I maintained the basic diabetic diet: lots of proteins and fats and not many carbs. I was still taking the same amount of insulin each day (about thirty-one to thirty-five units of long-lasting insulin), and I continued to exercise. My blood sugar levels were more or less the same as they had been when I was in college (my A1C was about 9.3%). Fortunately for me, some of the discipline that I'd learned over the past couple years stuck.

When I say that I took my insulin, I mean that I gave myself a shot. I was tired of having an insulin pump attached to my body 24/7, and I feel like I'm more aware of my diabetes without the pump, so I got rid of it and went back to traditional shots. I wanted to see how they worked for me after being on the pump for so many years. The shots were working, and my small lapses in discipline in my diet weren't all that serious. I was managing my diabetes better.

I spent a full year in India enjoying quality time with my family, visiting my grandparents, seeing old familiar sights, enjoying aspects of life that can only be found in India. I wasn't sure what I was going to do when I went back to the US, so I started toying with this or that idea. The one that was most interesting to me was the idea of working as a makeup artist. I'd always been told that I had a knack for applying my own makeup, and I sometimes gave my friends pointers. I also have a long creative streak, so I decided that makeup artistry was something that I might be able to pour myself into. I asked my sister to be my model, and she agreed to do her part to help me learn. After I had enough practice to boost my confidence, I approached several people about working as an apprentice. Two people agreed to work with me: a celebrity makeup artist and the head makeup artist at a salon. They were superb teachers, and I learned far more from them than I could have learned on my own. I grew to love the trade, and much of the stress that I'd brought from the US dissipated. I finally knew what I wanted to do for a living.

During that year in India, my relationship with Arjun continued to flourish. We talked over FaceTime every day, and we sent countless texts back and forth over the course of the year. In all that time, I never felt that our love for each waned. In fact, I felt closer to him than ever, which was ironic since we were about 7,700 miles apart. It became clear to me during my time in India that he was the man I wanted to spend the rest of my with. We both knew that this relationship was leading somewhere, and we talked about how good a match we were for each other and about the possibility of marriage. We are both traditional people, and we wanted to make sure that we had our families' blessings, so he came to India with his mother to discuss marriage with my family.

I was so incredibly happy to see him again after nearly a year of separation. We spent a month together, and we had a beautiful time. We went to dinners, met my family, and took long walks together. I was certain that he was the perfect man for me, and my family loved him too.

At one of the dinners that my parents hosted for us at a restaurant in Delhi, Arjun gave me the biggest surprise of my life. He walked into the restaurant with a huge bouquet of gorgeous flowers. After he set them on my table, he got down on one knee, presented me with a ring, and asked for my hand in marriage. And he did it all in front of my entire family. The eyes of every person in the room were full of tears, including mine. It was like a scene from a romantic movie, and it made me feel so special. And of course I said yes!

His proposal was in October of 2015, and we planned to get married in February of the following year, which meant that we had a lot of wedding arrangements to make in not much time. The venue, the music, the food and drinks, the flowers, the decorations, the guests, our wedding attire—the list goes on and on.

My life seemed perfect then. I'd been so down in the months before I left the US, but a little less than a year later, I'd reconnected with family and friends I hadn't seen in years, I'd finally found a career I knew I would adore, I spent a month sharing my family and my old life with the man I love, and, to top it all off, I got engaged. I was happier than I dared to hope I could ever be.

If there was a black mark on that period of my life, it was the small limp that I suddenly developed in the last couple days of Arjun's visit. I was pretty distracted by our engagement and by all the other wonderful things that were happening in my life, so I didn't think much of it, and neither did my family. When someone mentioned my limp, my family said that it was just, "Bainti being Bainti. She loves drama."

They were right about a lot things, but they couldn't have been more wrong about that limp.

FIVE

October of 2015 was the most significant month of my life. It was one of those cosmic turning points, where everything got flipped upside down. Bad became good and good became bad.

Just days after Arjun returned to the US, I woke and discovered that my legs felt weak. I wondered it if might have something to do with the limp I'd recently developed, but I really wasn't all that worried. My family's words were still ringing in my ears: "She loves drama." I figured that it was some mild condition that would clear up in a few days, and my family wasn't much concerned either. The consensus was that I'd be fine in no time.

Two days later, my sister and I had to go out of town for our cousin's birthday. We got up bright and early to catch a 5 a.m. train. At the train station, there was a small step to get up on the platform to board the train. When I tried to take that step, I couldn't lift my leg. My brain was giving my body commands, but my body was disobeying. My sister was already on the platform, and I didn't want to lose her, so I tried to take the step again. My leg didn't reply a second time, and I lost my balance and fell hard, twisting my ankle severely. I yelled for my sister, and she turned around and came running back to where I lay. My dad had just dropped us off at the train station and saw me fall. He jumped out of his car and rushed to my side. I tried to get up, but my legs were weak and I was in incredible pain. The trip to my cousin's house was obviously over for me, so my dad picked me up and carried me to his car. Because we all figured that I'd only sprained my ankle, my dad took me home so I could ice and elevate my foot. I popped a couple over-the-counter pain relievers, and I camped out on my bed for the day.

After a day of rest, the pain was still really bad, and I couldn't walk. I tried and tried to lift my legs, but the muscles wouldn't reply. It was as if there was a disconnect between my brain and my feet. Somewhere somehow the neural pathway was being disrupted. My parents, who thought it was just a sprain, told me that I'd be fine in a couple days, but I knew there was something very wrong with my body.

A couple days later, my legs were still weak and my ankle still hurt, so we went to an orthopedic specialist. It turned out that I hadn't just sprained my ankle; I'd torn a ligament. The doctor told me that I had to be in a cast for about a month and that I needed physical therapy if I hoped to be well enough to dance—or even to walk—at my wedding. It was November then, so I had a little more than three months to get healthy. I told myself that there was no way that I was going to postpone the wedding because of the injury and whatever ailment was causing the weakness in my legs, and I promised myself that I'd do everything in my power to get well soon. I wasn't going to disappoint Arjun or our families. I was going to work harder than I'd ever worked to get back on my feet.

For the next month, a physical therapist came to my home every day to do exercises with me to try to strengthen my legs, but nothing worked. So I pushed harder, convinced that I could will my legs back to health. They didn't respond though. In fact, things started to get worse. In addition to the weakness, the right side of my body went numb, all except my face. I also struggled to keep my balance. Now walking wasn't my only issue. Standing was becoming difficult for me as well. After a couple of weeks, my physical therapist recognized that I wasn't making any progress, and he suggested that I visit a doctor.

Sometime toward the end of November, my parents took me to see a neurologist in Delhi. He made me get all sorts of tests done, including an MRI and blood work. He also recommended that I get five sets of steroid treatments through an IV in order to help me walk again. We agreed to the treatment, and I received the steroid over a five day period. It did absolutely nothing for me, so we moved on to other options, to bigger hospitals with more doctors and fancier technology.

We visited just about every major hospital in Delhi: the Medanta Mediclinic, the Indraprastha Apollo Hospital, the Max Healthcare Institute. The hospitals were huge and impressive, but the treatment that I received there was no better than the treatment I'd received elsewhere. I'm no doctor, but I always thought it was strange that the neurologists I saw never even looked at my MRI scans. They only reviewed the reports from the physicians who had already seen me. I don't know if they were all just too busy to care or if they were trying not to step on the toes of other doctors, but I never got a new perspective, no matter how many neurologists I saw. Some of the doctors told me that I had diabetic neuropathy and that there was nothing they could do for me. Others told me that I had a problem with the nerves in my spine, and they wanted to do a spinal tap. The thought of a needle in my spine terrified me, especially since there was no guarantee that it would actually help in the long run. And one doctor told me that I had multiple sclerosis and that my life was going to be hard. That was the most horrifying possibility of them all. If I had MS, my life would never be the same.

Because the doctors in Delhi couldn't get to the bottom of the problem, we thought that we should try doctors in the US. We sent the reports to a doctor friend in California. He took a look at them, then handed them around to several of his colleagues. They all came to the same conclusion: everything seemed normal. Huh? In my book, paralysis is definitely not normal. We were all so confused.

While my parents and I tried to figure out what was happening with my legs, I updated Arjun in California daily about my health. He felt helpless, but he offered incredible emotional support during this tough period.

Around this time, one of my mother's friends suggested that I visit her doctor, who was a practitioner of holistic medicine. His name is Dr. Manik Hiranandani, and we made an appointment with him for the following week. I wasn't holding my breath that he'd succeed where all the other doctors had failed, but I was willing to visit anyone who might be able to help me in any way.

I knew right away that Dr. Manik wasn't like the other doctors. Before he even examined me, he reviewed my MRI scan, studying it diligently. Then he looked at all of my blood tests. In minutes he saw a pattern that all the other doctors had missed. He told me that I didn't have diabetic neuropathy or MS. He said that I had lead poisoning. He pulled up some information on his laptop and showed me a comparison of the symptoms of MS and the symptoms of lead poisoning. They were virtually identical. Could that really be the problem? Lead poisoning?

I wasn't sure if I should be ecstatic or terrified. I was happy to know that I didn't have an incurable, degenerative disease, but lead poisoning was a pretty serious diagnosis. At least I knew exactly what was wrong with me, and now we could focus on therapies that would help me heal.

Dr. Manik told me that I needed craniosacral therapy, which were adjustments to my spine, my neck, and my skull. He also gave me some exercises to do at home, which were meant to stretch my spine. I wasn't sure how spine adjustments were supposed to help me recover from lead poisoning, but I would have stood on my head and barked like a seal if I thought there was a chance that it would help me return me to full health.

We visited his office twice for craniosacral adjustments, and felt lighter instantly. I'll admit that I was skeptical about his treatments at first, but after just two visits, I definitely felt better, much lighter on my feet, although I did still have numbness and weakness in my legs. Dr. Manik had a clinic in Southern India, so he had to head south after only two treatments, but he encouraged me to try other forms of therapy, including acupressure and exercise.

My mom found an acupressurist who could come to our home and do treatments on me every day. He did acupressure on my feet and my hands, and I did all the exercises that Dr. Manik recommended. Sure enough, I started to regain strength and mobility, little by little, day by day. My body eventually became mine again. When my brain told my legs to lift or to move, they listened. I felt like a parent who was finally connecting with her child after some difficult teenage years.

I was overjoyed that I was clawing my way back to health, but I was especially happy to know that my stubborn body wouldn't spoil my wedding. As long as my healing continued on its upward trend, I was going to be able stand and dance and not worry about Arjun's disappointment in his bride's inability to stand on her own two feet.

SIX

I got married on February 13, 2016. It was the happiest—and the luckiest—day of my life.

Thanks to the adjustments I'd received at Dr. Manik's office, the acupressure treatments, and the exercises I did on my own at home, I was able to walk properly the day we got married in Delhi. I even managed to dance, although I was a little stiff. Nobody seemed to mind though. Arjun and I had a lovely time, and my guests all seemed quite pleased.

Arjun—my husband!—and I stayed in a hotel in Delhi for four days after our wedding. On our third day there, I started getting some weakness in my right leg again. We were leaving the next day for our honeymoon in Koh Samui, Thailand, so I did all my physical therapy exercises so I wouldn't miss out on any of the fun we planned to have. Stretching, acupressure, leg lifts—I did it all, hoping I could prevent a regression that would interfere with our lives. Unfortunately for us both, the treatments didn't help. I didn't regain any of the strength in my right leg, and I actually lost some of the mobility I'd worked so hard to recover before my wedding.

Arjun and I talked about possibly postponing our honeymoon so I could work on my mobility, but in the end we decided that it was best to go and to make the best of the situation. The purpose of a honeymoon is to share uninterrupted time with your new spouse. I know that many people spend a good chunk of their honeymoons kayaking down rivers or taking in the scenery on a zip line, but that's all secondary to other activities like sharing breakfast in bed or watching the sunset from your hotel balcony. I'd have to skip some of the outdoorsy stuff, but we would still share a beautiful experience because we would be together, united in matrimony, beginning our adventure as a married couple. I also hoped that if I continued with my exercises, I might be fine. Those exercises had helped before my wedding, and I was hopeful that they could help again.

So off we went to Koh Samui, excited about everything that lay in front of us. Our flight arrived about 10:00 in the morning, and we went directly from the airport to our hotel to check in. I loved everything about Koh Samui. It was so beautiful, so green. It was an island bursting with life, and I felt energized by the vibrance of the place.

A day into our honeymoon, my legs got worse. I did all the exercises I was supposed to do, but nothing helped. My legs became very weak, and I had a hard time walking without support. I had to hold on to someone or something so I wouldn't fall, which I started doing far too often. In fact, I was falling and getting hurt so frequently that we had to request the use of a wheelchair. The hotel allowed us to use one, and Arjun had to wheel me around. When we went out to do touristy things, we had to take that wheelchair along. I did my best to put a happy face on the situation, but it was difficult not to feel let down by the state of my health.

Arjun did his best to make our honeymoon seem as normal as possible. When we talked or texted with any of our family or friends, we didn't tell them about what was really happening. I was scared and confused, and we did everything we could to hide my weakness. We took no pictures that showed that I was having trouble walking or that I had to use a wheelchair. I didn't like seeing myself in that state, and I didn't want that wheelchair immortalized in my honeymoon pictures. That was one memory I didn't want to keep forever.

We had some beautiful experiences, but I felt so bad for Arjun. I apologized to him again and again, but he reassured me that he was happy so long as he was around me, whether I was standing at his side or sitting in a wheelchair in front of him. I wouldn't have married him if I hadn't been certain that he had a kind soul and a caring heart, but this was just more proof that I'd found the perfect man.

We tried to make the best of our time together in Koh Samui, but the weakness in my legs eventually became so debilitating that we decided to go to the hospital so I could get checked out. I had absolutely no eye-foot coordination, especially in my right leg. I couldn't move it at all, not even a little bit. They admitted me into the hospital for observation, but the doctors didn't have any answers for me. Mine was one of those cases that you see on a medical mystery show on the Discovery Channel. Lots of weird symptoms; not many reasonable explanations.

My experiences in hospitals made me acutely aware of the limits of the understanding of the medical profession. When I was younger, I imagined that doctors had all the answers when it came to illness and disease, but what I discovered as an adult is that doctors are only as good as their training and their experiences, both of which are limited. They go to medical school for four years, where they learn something about a lot of different potential health problems, but there are aspects of health that they really don't touch on. I know that diet is one of those blind spots in the medical profession. The foods that we eat have a profound impact on our health—take it from a diabetic—but when non-diabetics like Arjun walk into a doctor's office, the doctor rarely asks him what sorts of foods he eats. That seems so counterintuitive to me. Shouldn't that be one of the first questions a doctor asks? They have you step on the scale so they can check your weight, but then they don't ask about the role that food might be playing in determining that weight.

I guess what I'm trying to say is that you should always bring your critical-thinking skills with you when you go to a clinic or a hospital. You have to be your own chief health-care advocate. Unless you've studied medicine, you probably don't understand much about anatomy or about biochemical processes, so you shouldn't trick yourself into believing that you know more than they do about the human body. But they don't know how it feels to be in *your* body the way that you do. You know your aches and pains, your twitches and flutters. And they also don't have to live with their mistakes the way that you do. A misdiagnosis might lead to a couple sleepless nights for the doctor, but it could lead to a lifetime of suffering for you. Be respectful of a doctor's knowledge and experiences, but don't be a pushover. If something about what the doctor is saying doesn't feel right to you, make sure you ask a lot of questions. If the doctor can't or won't answer your questions, then get a second, third, or even fourth opinion, or get out of there, as long as leaving won't put your life or the lives of others in immediate danger. You're the boss of your body. Don't ever forget that.

I stayed in that hospital in Koh Samui for a day. The doctors told me that they didn't have any answers for me, and they suggested that I visit a hospital in Bangkok, where there were more experienced physicians. We thanked them for their advice, then I signed myself out.

After we left the hospital, Arjun and I talked it over, and we decided that our best option was to cut our honeymoon short and head back to India. We would gather our belongings in Delhi, say goodbye to my parents and the rest of my family, and then fly to the US. We would figure out our next move at home.

SEVEN

After our honeymoon, Arjun and I returned to California to begin our new lives as a married couple. To save up money to pay for my health-care expenses and possibly to buy a house someday, we decided to move in with his parents, my in-laws. They're very loving, and I'm blessed to be a part of their family.

Our first priority was obviously my health. Nothing else matters all that much if you don't have your health. I know he didn't mind pushing me around in a wheelchair, but that wasn't the life I wanted for him or for myself.

Because I'd had type 1 since 2002, I guessed that I must have diabetic neuropathy, a type of nerve damage that affects your ability to use your hands and feet. In the weeks immediately following our return to the US, Arjun took me to one doctor after another. They ran countless tests on me to rule out this and that. In the end, they delivered the worst possible diagnosis: multiple sclerosis. Another autoimmune disease? Really? As if diabetes wasn't enough already, now I had MS. I cried for most of the rest of that day.

Eventually I wiped away my tears and started doing a

little digging on the Internet. What I found was somewhat heartening. While there was a chance that I could become bedridden or wheelchair bound in less than fifteen years after the onset of symptoms, my chances were better than fifty-fifty that I'd be able to get around on my own. According to the research studies I read, about 60% of MS sufferers can walk without assistance—so long as they take their prescribed medications.

My doctor wanted me to start on a medication regimen immediately, so he sent me to my local pharmacy, where I picked up a bottle of pills that were meant to reduce the inflammation they said was weakening my central nervous system. The medication wasn't a cure—there is no cure for MS—but it would slow the progression of the disease and give me back some of my mobility. I hated that I had to take more medications every day on top of insulin. I just didn't feel right taking the pills, and I didn't want to depend on medication all my life, so I waited, debating whether or not I should take them. After a week, my numbness got worse and walking became more difficult, so I gave in and took the pills.

My first day on my new meds was really tough. I broke out into hives, and I was nauseated all day. My doctors told me that those were normal side effects, but their reassurances didn't do anything to make me feel any less miserable.

That night, Arjun and I went to a friend's house. After we arrived, the nausea became horrible, so I excused myself to check my blood sugar level. I assumed that it was low, but it came back at 87, which is normal. I returned to the dinner party with Arjun and our friends, and just minutes later, I blacked out. Arjun gave me a glucose injection that brought me back to consciousness. I was able to sit up, but our night was obviously done.

We decided to see a specialist in the days after that fainting episode. Wanting treatment from the best of the best, we went to the Stanford Medical Center in Palo Alto, not far from where we lived. The doctor I saw there also diagnosed me with MS, and he said that he wanted me to start taking weekly injections on top of the pills I was already taking. He told me that if I didn't start on the medications that he prescribed, I could be wheelchair bound in the next three to six months. He told me that I should prepare to lose control of my body and that I should get used to being dependent. He painted a very bleak picture of my future.

Arjun and I were quiet during the drive home from Stanford. I didn't know what to say to him, and I'm sure he didn't know what to say to me. We'd only been married for a few weeks to that point, and here we were learning that I could be stuck in a wheelchair for the rest of my life, starting in as little as a quarter of a year. Our lives would be so much more restricted than we ever imagined they would be. We would never hike in Yosemite or scuba dive off the coast of Australia. I wouldn't be able to play tag with our children or teach them how to swim. Maybe Arjun wouldn't even want to have kids with me. Maybe he would be too overwhelmed with the additional responsibilities of caring for someone who couldn't walk on her own, and he wouldn't want to take on the added responsibility of raising children as well. It seemed like the life we'd just started building for ourselves was crashing down around us. It felt as though we'd just put the roof on our dream house and a tornado had come through and smashed it all to smithereens.

At home we went straight upstairs to figure out what to do next. We talked for hours, carefully weighing each option. I hated the idea of taking yet another heavy medication for the rest of my life, but I wasn't exactly in love with the prospect of spending my days in a wheelchair. I also wondered if the side effects were worth the benefits. Who knew what all those drugs would do to my body? But I did know that none of those medications would cure the disease. The doctors told me that my body would still deteriorate if I took medicine. It would only slow the process. Arjun shared my concerns and my worries, and he suggested that we look into natural doctors to see if there was anything they could do to help me regain my mobility without the drugs. Dr. Manik in India was a holistic healer, and he'd helped me get back onto my feet before my wedding. Maybe we could find a similar doctor in the Bay Area.

We started researching naturopathic doctors around the area. After talking to several of them, we found one who was confident that she could help me. Over the phone, she promised that I'd begin feeling better immediately after she started caring for me. I loved her energy and her certainty, so I made an appointment for the next week. I thought that seeing her would be well worth the risk. The worst that could happen would be that her treatment wouldn't do anything for me, and we'd be back at square one. If that happened, we could just move on to the next doctor.

At our appointment the following week, I shared my medical history with her. After listening carefully, she told me that she wanted me to start a food avoidance treatment immediately, right there in her office at that first appointment. She pulled out some vials that contained food from the categories I was supposed to avoid, then she performed acupuncture on me for about thirty minutes while I held the vials. I was then to go home and stay away from those foods at all costs. And that didn't mean that I just wasn't supposed to eat the foods. I also couldn't touch or smell them. I basically wasn't supposed to be around any air molecules that originated from the foods I had to avoid. This wasn't going to be easy.

What that meant in practical terms was that while I was doing the treatments, which lasted between twenty-four and forty hours, I couldn't leave my room at all or come into contact with anyone, including Arjun, who might have been around the foods. I couldn't open the windows in my room, and I either had to prepare my food in advance or ask for someone to make it for me. It wasn't just a trial for me; Arjun and my in-laws also had to make sacrifices. Because I couldn't even be in the same house with the foods I was supposed to avoid, they had to remove all traces of the foods from their cabinets and their refrigerator. And they had to prepare a lot of meals for me. They were tremendously accommodating, but I felt guilty about asking them to make those sacrifices for me.

In addition to avoiding certain food categories, I also had to keep a log of every meal I ate so the doctor could later determine how my body was reacting to the treatments. On top of that, I had drink a Chinese herb mixture that tasted horrible. I had to put it in my tea so I could bear the bitterness. I drank it twice a day, plugging my nose as I swallowed it. I told myself that it was a small price to pay if it could help me avoid that wheelchair.

By far the most difficult treatment was mineral avoidance. For two days I wasn't supposed to drink or touch any water that wasn't distilled, which meant that I couldn't take a shower or brush my teeth with water from the tap. I had to buy gallons and gallons of distilled water for drinking, bathing, and brushing. Arjun even had to bathe in distilled water before he entered the room after he came home from work. As with every other avoidance treatment, he was my rock. He never complained once.

I wish I could say that every avoidance treatment went as planned, but of course that wouldn't be the truth. While I was doing the mineral avoidance treatment, I went to the bathroom one morning and stepped on a small drop of water on the floor. Almost immediately I developed a horrendous headache, and red, itchy patches broke out all over my body. I had to start the treatment over again, and that was mentally exhausting.

The doctor had stated very clearly that I'd begin to feel better almost immediately after I started the treatments, but I didn't feel better at all. In fact, I actually started to feel worse in many ways. I developed numbness and tingling, which came and went throughout the day, in both of my legs and in my hands. I also got terrible intermittent nerve pain, usually around the same places I'd developed numbness. As a result, I had a lot of trouble walking. There were times when I had to hold on to the wall so I wouldn't fall; there were other times when I couldn't even stand on my own. Sometimes I had to crawl on top of a chair or some other piece of furniture to push myself up. Then there was the pain at night. It woke me from sleep three or four times every night, and that made me feel tired all day, which didn't do my mental health any favors. The lack of sleep made me paranoid about everything. If I slept wrong on my hand and caused it to fall asleep, I woke convinced that my disease was getting worse and that I was another day closer to a wheelchair. That paranoia became confusion and depression. No one seemed to have any answers, and I couldn't see any solution in sight. Whenever I thought about my health, I cried, and the more I cried, the more I thought about my health. It was a vicious circle that was quickly spiraling out of control. This was the lowest point of my life.

To help me cope with the stress and the depression, Arjun suggested that I start using CBD, which stands for cannabidiol, a naturally occurring cannabinoid found in cannabis, also known as marijuana. Prior to his suggestion, I'd heard that CBD was something of a wonder drug, but I was always doubtful because of the propaganda that had been spread about cannabis during the US government's war on drugs. But I was desperate for a solution, and I was willing to try anything that could possibly help, so I did some research. The more I dug into articles and blogs, the more encouraged I felt. There were so many success stories floating out there about how useful the drug had been in helping with this or that symptom. Before long, my fears had abated, and I was ready to give CBD a shot. More than anything, I wanted a way out of the depression. I hoped that the drug would help me get my mind in the right place. If I could recover my mental health, I could figure out what my next step should be to recover my physical health, or at least to minimize my symptoms. I wanted my life to be as normal as possible.

I visited a local dispensary with Arjun, and we bought some CBD drops and a CBD/THC (one-to-one ratio) vape pen cartridge. The employee at the dispensary recommended that I take the CBD/THC cartridge because they're supposed to work better in tandem. I took the drops under my tongue every morning and every night, and I inhaled the contents of the cartridge a couple times a day. After a week, I felt a little better, and I increased my dosage. The results were really promising.

The biggest change that I noticed after using cannabis

for only a couple weeks was that I was no longer waking up in the middle of the night in excruciating pain, and I started sleeping through the night. I also got control of my anxiety and my depression. If I ever felt the darkness sneaking up on me, I pulled out my vape pen and got some nearly instant relief. I hate to sound like a drug addict who could only cope with hardship through self-medication, but the truth is that cannabis was and still is incredibly helpful to my mental health. It also made a huge difference in the way that stress manifested in my body. Because my body seemed to be falling apart one piece at a time, I was unconsciously stiffening muscles everywhere. I was constantly anticipating worse and worse news, and my body had been tense for months. Cannabis helped me loosen up in a way that nothing else ever had.

EIGHT

I know I've sung Arjun's praises in earlier pages, but I want to take a moment here to really brag about my incredible husband. Part of the reason I'd become so depressed over the past year was because I was worried that I was a burden to Arjun. Newlyweds are typically so smitten with each other that they spend every waking moment in their first year of marriage soaking in their new spouses, but our first year was spent addressing my physical and mental health issues. A less devoted man than Arjun might have turned tail when it became clear that we weren't going to have a typical newlywed relationship, but that's not Arjun's style. He was so supportive during my lowest days that I sometimes cried in appreciation of his kindness. Whenever he was around me, he tried to encourage me to put my woes out of my mind for a while and enjoy life. He worked hard to make me smile or laugh, and he usually succeeded. When he came home after working all day, we cozied up on the couch and watched comedy movies together so I wouldn't have a choice but to laugh. And he constantly pushed me to get out of the house so I wouldn't sit around feeling that there was something wrong with me or that I didn't deserve to be out there with our friends living my life. We went out almost every weekend, usually to dinner, but sometimes also to bars. Some nights we went out by ourselves; other nights we hung out with our friends. Whatever the particulars, our nights out were always fun. Arjun has an infectious lust for life, and whenever I'm around him, I can't help but to pick up on his positive energy. He makes me a better person, and I don't think I'm exaggerating when I say that I have the best husband in the world.

When our first anniversary rolled around, I became very reflective. Thinking back on our first year of marriage, my impulse was to feel guilty for putting Arjun through the wringer, but he wouldn't let me. On the weekend of our anniversary, he took me on a romantic getaway to Half Moon Bay. As we were driving to our hotel on our first day there, Arjun told me that he had one request: he didn't want me to mention my health once all weekend. He told me that he thought I was perfect just the way I was, and he didn't want me to beat myself up over my problems. I gladly granted him his request, and we didn't bring up any of my health issues all weekend. It was absolutely wonderful, and I'll forever cherish the memories we made there.

Once we returned from our anniversary weekend, we got back into my food avoidance routine. To that point, I'd successfully finished about twenty tests, and I had thirteen more to go. I was pretty frustrated with the whole process by then because I wasn't seeing any positive results. In fact, it seemed to me that I was actually moving backwards. My legs were still numb from the thigh down, and my hands were also starting to lose sensation and beginning to tremble uncontrollably. Before my hands went numb, I'd tried to distract my mind from my disease by doing freelance makeup work, but after I lost coordination, I could no longer do it. Doing makeup every day would have been really good for my mental health, but that wasn't in my cards right then.

I was beginning to doubt very seriously that the treatments I was receiving were going to help me return to health. At an appointment with the doctor who had prescribed the food-avoidance treatments, I reminded her that she'd told me that I'd see immediate results once she took over my care, but I'd made no progress after nearly six months. I asked her a ton of questions about the direction the treatment was headed, and I got the feeling she was a little confused. I knew then that it was time for me to start looking for another doctor.

I was feeling pretty low about my health again, and Arjun recognized the signs of depression, so he told me that he wanted to take me out for the day so I could get out of my head. We went to a mall to do some window shopping and to get a treat at the food court. While we were walking around, I came across a chiropractor's booth. His name was Dr. Fawaz Albadani. Arjun insisted that I take a minute to talk with the chiropractor, thinking that he might be able to do something for me. The doctor suggested that I come to his office to get an X-ray of my spine. All the other doctors I'd seen at that point had taken X-rays of my legs, but none of them had ever taken images of my back. I was curious to see if there might be something wrong with my spine, so I agreed to come to his office.

After Dr. Fawaz took X-rays, he told me that I didn't have any curvature of the spine that could result in a pinched nerve that would cause numbness, tingling, and weakness. He suggested that I get some chiropractic adjustments, and I agreed to let him work on me. He performed a number of treatments on my neck and spine, and we did a variety of exercises both at his office and at home. The exercises, which were sometimes brutally painful, stretched my spine and loosened the muscles of my body. The most excruciating exercise involved a foam roller that I used on my legs. I hated those exercises, but the agony was well worth it in the end.

After daily adjustments and treatments for three months, I was able to walk normally again. The natural curve of my spine also returned. My numbness and tingling came and went, but overall I was feeling better than I'd felt in more than a year. I was amazed by what Dr. Fawaz had done for my body, and I felt so fortunate that I'd bumped into him at the mall.

Eventually Dr. Fawaz told me that he wanted me to consider coming to a dinner seminar that he was hosting to discuss autoimmune diseases. I was usually in and out of Dr. Fawaz's office in less than half an hour, but our appointment lasted about three hours that day. He talked extensively about the nationwide network of medical practitioners he'd recently joined. The network included doctors from various medical fields, and they were all committed to treating patients naturally. Arjun and I were excited by what he shared, and we told him that we'd both attend the dinner.

At the seminar, Dr. Fawaz spoke at length about his general philosophy of healing. He believes that the body has the power to heal itself, but the key to effective treatment is different for each person. He believes that a treatment plan should be personalized, based on what a person's test results show, and he focuses on fixing the underlying problem rather than simply mitigating the symptoms or managing the disease. Why take medications for life when you can solve the problem that necessitates the medications? I was intrigued by what he had to say about helping people return to full health, and I smiled throughout his discussion.

Dr. Fawaz also talked a lot about leaky gut syndrome, which he believes is the cause of a variety of conditions, including multiple sclerosis, autism, fibromyalgia, chronic fatigue syndrome, thyroid abnormalities, migraines, and many others. According to Dr. Fawaz, the intestinal wall usually blocks the passage of bacteria and toxins, but if the intestines become more permeable (in other words, "leaky"), bacteria and toxins can pass from the intestines into the bloodstream, which can cause inflammation and provoke a reaction from the body's immune system. That reaction is the source of many of the ailments that plague people like me.

While at the seminar, I met a woman who'd brought her sister with her to convince her to start Dr. Fawaz's treatments. The woman was a type 2 diabetic, and she'd been dealing with horrendous nerve pain for years before she met Dr. Fawaz. Her pain was so severe that she found it difficult to walk most days. She'd tried every medication known to humankind, and none of them work. She'd almost given up hope of leading a pain-free life when she met Dr. Fawaz. After just a couple months of treatment, she felt significantly better. Much of her pain was gone, and she had no problem walking any more. Now she wanted to share the benefits of his treatments with her sister, and with everyone else she knew who was suffering from some lingering physical ailment.

Arjun and I really liked the seminar. To me, this was such a novel way of approaching healthcare, but it also seemed so intuitive. Our bodies are each unique. Everyone has different bacteria biomes living inside them, so it makes sense that each body would need a different treatment to address health problems. We walked away full of hope, convinced that Dr. Fawaz was going to be the person who'd help me get my health back on track.

I had an appointment with him the following day, and we started right in on treatments. The first step was to get blood work done. The next step was to test for food sensitivities, which would measure my body's immune response to a number of foods. He explained that when a food triggers your immune system, it causes inflammation, which leads to disease. Once I had my food sensitivity results, for the next three months I was supposed to avoid the foods that cause my body's immune system to kick in. I was also supposed to take certain natural herbal supplements, which varied from person to person, depending on the results of the blood tests. After three months, I could re-introduce those foods back into my diet. If I noticed any physical response to the food, whether it was an upset stomach or a skin rash, I needed to continue avoiding those foods. But if my body didn't respond negatively, I could bring those foods back into my diet.

I was incredibly excited to start Dr. Fawaz's treatment. I loved that his plan was tailor-made for each individual, and I really appreciated Dr. Fawaz's obvious concern for my health. He has an amazing bedside manner, and he seemed eager to help me overcome my healthcare problems.

As much as Dr. Fawaz supported me, he still came in a distant second to Arjun. My husband was always my number one, and this was no exception. To show his solidarity with me and to make sure I didn't feel alone—and to improve his overall health—Arjun had his blood tested when I had mine tested. He wanted to endure everything I endured, to prove to me that I could always count on him, not that I needed him to prove anything to me. He'd already shown me countless times how reliable and supportive he is.

NINE

In May of 2017, my parents flew out from India to visit us because they were concerned about all my health issues. I hadn't seen them since our wedding in February of the previous year, and I missed them terribly. I'd wanted to go to India to visit them, but we didn't want to interrupt my treatments. They came out to see us instead.

We had a wonderful time together, and they helped me forget about my health concerns while they were visiting. They wanted details about everything we were doing to address my problems, so I filled them in on all that had transpired over the past several months. When I told them about Dr. Fawaz's food sensitivity test, they got their tests done too as a way of showing their support. That was a very sweet gesture, and I appreciated it more than I could say. The week that they were here flew by, and I was sad to see them go.

I got the food sensitivity results back a week after they left. It turned out that I was sensitive to seventeen different foods, including eggs, mushrooms, rice, yeast, and black and white pepper, to name just a few. In order to start the treatment, I had to become gluten and dairy free, which meant that I had to cut out a lot of my favorite foods. This was going to be a challenging few months, but then I was already used to challenges. If I could manage to hobble around on two almost-useless legs for so long, I could manage this. Giving up bread and cheese was a small price to pay to avoid ending up in a wheelchair. One thing I didn't have to give up was CBD, which I regularly used—with Dr. Fawaz's blessing—as a substitute for some of the ingredients I could no longer use when cooking.

The first three months of the treatment were difficult. Avoiding seventeen different types of food at once means that you have to get creative in the kitchen. Two months into the treatment though, I noticed a significant improvement in my mental and physical health. I was happier than I'd been in quite a while, and I had far more energy than I'd had prior to beginning the treatment. I still had some numbness and weakness in my legs, but I felt lighter on my feet. The numbness and weakness in my hands also vanished, and I could easily write once again. Of all the treatments I'd had over the past year, this one was by far the most effective. We still weren't finished with the treatments yet, but so far Dr. Fawaz was looking like a miracle worker.

When I met with Dr. Fawaz at the three-month point, I talked with him about extending the food-restriction treatment for another three months. Avoiding all those foods was obviously working wonders on my body, and it didn't make sense to me to discontinue a plan of action that was showing results. Dr. Fawaz thought it was a good idea to push on with the food restrictions as well, but he did ask me to get a stool test done to find out if I had any inflammation or infections in my gut. When I got the results back, he put me on herbal supplements to counter some toxic bacteria and a yeast infection, and it was clear that it was best to continue avoiding those foods.

After another three months of restrictions, Dr. Fawaz said that I could start reintroducing some of those seventeen foods back into my diet. I started with mushrooms, yeast, and black and white pepper. He also said that I could reintroduce gluten and dairy into my diet if I wanted, but he suggested that I continue to avoid them if possible. I told him that I preferred to cut them out of my diet altogether. I was convinced that they were major culprits in my illnesses.

I was a bit worried that my body would regress, but Dr. Fawaz assured me that I could return to the restrictions immediately if he saw any indications that the foods were causing me to become ill again. Fortunately for me, and for my taste buds, my body didn't react poorly to any of the foods I reintroduced into my diet. The combination of cannabis and dietary restrictions was giving me back my health and my happiness. Each day that passed, I felt a little better. My blood sugar level was improving every day, and I was taking less insulin. The numbness in my legs was almost entirely gone, and I could stand on my own with no problem. I had more energy than I remember ever having, and I was able to go on long walks Arjun again.

I did have one minor setback around this time, but Dr. Fawaz helped me with that as well. One of the things Dr. Fawaz had told me before we began his treatment was that when I started treating my body right, it would release various toxins from various places. He was right about that. I constantly had to rush to the bathroom during those months. When I woke up one morning with a swollen left eye, I assumed that it was a sign of more toxins being excreted from my body. It seemed like a stye, so I kept a warm compress on it for the day. The next morning it was so swollen and painful that I couldn't open it. I went to my primary care physician, and she told me that I had shingles. She prescribed a medication that had a steroid as a primary ingredient. Because I hate taking medications, I didn't get the prescription filled. Instead, I went to Dr. Fawaz's office. I asked him if I could heal my shingles naturally, and he told me about some homeopathic remedies, which I started immediately. I applied a CBD salve on my eye to help with the often-unbearable pain. My nerves felt like they were being yanked out of my body. After fifteen days of natural remedies at home, including cannabis, my eye was back to normal. I had no more pain, and I had absolutely no scarring. It was like it never happened, which, again, just goes to show you the power of nature.

People who have known me for years were amazed by the progress I'd made that year. More than one person told me that I seemed like a totally different person. When they asked me what my secret was, I told them that I was finally starting to understand my body. It had certain needs in order to function efficiently, and I was just now figuring out how to give it what it needed.

I've been hearing for years that you just have to eat the right foods in order to stay healthy. That sounds simple enough, but it turns out that it's somewhat complicated because the "right" foods differ from person to person. Gluten might be fine for one person, but it could be toxic to someone else. One person might remain perfectly healthy by eating cheese every day, but cheese might cause another person all sorts of health complications. The biggest problem with the idea of the "right" foods is that it often isn't clear when a food is having a negative impact on someone's body. Sometimes the symptoms of food allergies are obvious: rashes, constricted breathing, an elevated heart rate. But a lot of people don't have such obvious reactions to foods, and they continue to eat foods that are toxic to their bodies. They slowly poison themselves, and when a serious disease crops up as a result of the long-term damage caused by the toxins, they rush to a doctor and get prescriptions for medications that do absolutely nothing to address the underlying cause of the disease. To heal the body, you must understand the body, and you'll never get that understanding unless you see a doctor who grasps the contribution that diet makes in maintaining health.

I felt great by the end of 2017, and I decided that in addition to the other foods I was avoiding, I also wanted to cut out meat. I was never one for red meat, but I did enjoy chicken and seafood a couple times a week. I loved the way that eating healthy made me feel, and I wondered if I would feel even better if I went vegetarian. I thought that it was an experiment worth trying, so I started researching a lot of plant-based diets and watching a variety of documentaries. Listening to the success stories told by other people motivated me to make the leap.

It took me about a month to get used to not eating meat, but in the end it proved to be a very successful experiment. I feel better than I've probably ever felt. I'd always been the sickly child, but now I feel like I can climb mountains and run marathons. I haven't tried either one yet, but at least I know that I could perform those feats of strength and endurance if I chose to. I no longer fear for my health. Instead, I feel tremendous love for my body because I finally have the body I've always wanted, the body that allows me to do anything that tickles my fancy. I love this new way of living.

I wanted to see exactly how my diet had affected my body's chemistry, so I visited my endocrinologist to get some lab work done. I was especially curious to check my A1C blood glucose and my thyroid peroxidase antibody levels. When I sat down with the doctor and told him exactly what I'd done to improve my health over the past half year, he frowned and told me that I was making a serious mistake. Because I was diabetic, he argued, I needed to be eating meat, which was, in his opinion, an essential source of protein. He said that he was sure that my A1C level would still be high and that my thyroid peroxidase antibody level would be worse than ever. He wanted me back on the insulin pump immediately, before we even did the lab work. He was so convinced that I was on the wrong path that he was willing to prescribe medication to me before he saw my results. Fortunately for me, I was wise to the ways of doctors by then, and I flat out refused to go back on the pump, especially not before seeing my labs.

When the results came back, my faith in Dr. Fawaz's abilities was completely vindicated. After a year of following his dietary restrictions, cutting dairy and meat, and adding cannabis to virtually everything I ate, my A1C level had dropped to 7.2%, which was lower than it had been for as long as I've been having my blood tested. As a result of that incredible improvement, I only have to take half as much insulin as I'd been taking before (fifteen units of long-lasting insulin). My thyroid peroxidase antibody level dropped from 490 IU/mL in 2016 to 130 IU/mL. At 130, my thyroid peroxidase antibody count is still high, but a drop of 360 is an incredible leap forward for me. That's a huge improvement through natural medicine rather than through pharmaceuticals. All of my other blood work came back in the healthy range as well, and the results of another stool test were also good. The cherry on top was the twenty-five pounds I'd shed over the previous year. And I think it's important to note that I wasn't following the "diabetic diet." I was eating carbs, but carbs don't make my blood sugar spike now.

Inside and out, I'm now as healthy as I've ever been. I'm no longer the sick girl. I've never felt so normal in all my life, and I couldn't be happier.

EPILOGUE

I've been eating the right foods for my body for about fifteen months now, and I've had no health issues in all that time. All my numbers are better than they've been in ages, my mental health is great, and my relationships have flourished. That's especially true of my marriage to Arjun. My battle against disease has made our bond incredibly tight, and in a weird way I'm glad that we went through that struggle together early on in our marriage because it made us stronger and brought us closer. Dr. Fawaz's treatment has also helped Arjun become healthier, not that he was in poor health to begin with. And like me, he says that he has never felt better.

Since I started eating the right food for my body, I feel like I've been given a new life. From as far back as I can remember, I've been dependent on other people for help. My mom, my dad, my doctors, my school nurses, my relatives, my in-laws, my husband—the list of supporters goes on and on. For all but the past year and a half of my life, I've needed a team of allies to help me function in the world. But now I feel like I'm in control of my health and my life for the first time. I determine what foods I eat, which determines how I feel. I know that I've still got that amazing circle of supporters if anything should ever go wrong with my health, but it's nice to know that they're just a safety net now. I'm not dependent on them for every little thing every day. So to all those who have helped me so much over the years, I want to express my deepest gratitude for all your love and support. But I also want you to know that I can handle it from here.

Some people have told me that my story is inspirational, but I think that people are giving me too much credit when they say such a thing. Dr. Fawaz is the real hero of this story. If I hadn't bumped into him at, of all places, a mall, I might be in a wheelchair right now. He did precisely what a doctor is supposed to do: he helped my body and my spirit heal. He gave me hope for a better future, one that doesn't involve Arjun pushing me around in a wheelchair. It seems to me that the word "healer" is a more appropriate word to describe Dr. Fawaz than the word "doctor." I'm certainly no expert on the state of medicine in this country, or in any country for that matter, but based on my experiences with physicians over the past couple decades, I've seen that far too many doctors don't do a lot of healing. They seem to manage diseases rather than to work to prevent them in the first place or to solve the underlying problems that cause them. That's not healing. That's symptom mitigation, which isn't the ideal approach for patients. Taking medication is obviously better than going without and suffering needlessly, but that's a very distant second to helping patients make changes that eliminate the need for medication.

I feel that a lot of the doctors I've seen both in the US and in India are stuck in a mindset that limits their ability to maximize the impact they have on the lives of their patients.

I think the medical profession needs to do some soul-searching. It takes time for a doctor to get to know a patient, to understand fully all the factors that are contributing to a patient's health or illness. If your doctor is making you feel like you're on an assembly line, then it might be time for you to start hunting for another one.

I know this is news to some doctors, but doctors aren't gods. They're people just like you and me, and it's important that you remember that the person in that white lab coat doesn't know everything. Don't blindly follow the advice of any doctor, no matter how intelligent or experienced that person might be. Make sure that you do your homework and investigate all possible avenues. You are your own best health advocate, and if you're not willing to put in the time to understand your body, then you might not get the care you need.

And that's really why I wrote this book: to help other people who might be fighting a battle like the one I fought for so many years. A lifestyle change is obviously not going to solve every medical condition, but I'm willing to go out on a limb and say that every medical condition can be improved at least somewhat by making changes to your lifestyle. And some conditions can be drastically improved if not completely cured by making smart choices about your health. I realize how difficult change is though. Being healthy definitely takes a lot of work, but the rewards are incalculable. For me, giving up some of the foods I love means that I'll be able to run with my future children at the park and swim with them in the ocean. For me, the right choice is obvious, and I know that someday my future self is going to thank me for making that decision today.

APPENDIX

A Word on Plants

Nearly 45% of the US has some chronic disease, which is an ongoing, generally incurable illnesses or condition, including heart disease, cancer, and diabetes. According to the American Heart Association, one in three children and adults are considered obese in the US. Approximately 30% of the deaths in the US are caused by a cardiovascular-related disease. An estimated twenty-three million adults in the US have diabetes, and about eighty million are considered pre-diabetic. Sadly, the numbers are rising.

Meat is a rich source of beneficial nutrients, such as protein, B vitamins, iron, and zinc, but red meat can also contain high amounts of saturated fat, and processed meats can be high in sodium. Plants are rich sources of nutrients like vitamins, minerals, fiber, and proteins that are important for good health. Eating a plant-based diet has been linked to a lowered risk and, in some cases, even a reversal of chronic diseases such as diabetes inflammations, cancers, and heart disease. The major benefits for patients who decide to start a plant-based diet are the possibility of reducing the number of medications they take to treat a variety of chronic conditions, lowering body weight, decreasing the risk of cancer, and reducing the risk of death from heart disease. Numerous recent studies have clearly shown that people whose diets include a large intake of plant-based foods tend to have a lower risk of chronic diseases.

A plant-based diet isn't an all-or-nothing proposition. It's a way of life that can be tailored to each individual. It may be especially beneficial for those with obesity, type 2 diabetes, high blood pressure, lipid disorders, or cardiovascular disease. A registered dietitian should be part of the healthcare team that designs a plant-based diet for patients with chronic disease, especially if multiple medications are involved. Depending on the underlying conditions, patients with chronic disease who take multiple medications need close monitoring of low blood sugar levels, low blood pressure, or rapid weight loss. In some cases, such as mine, the need for certain medications can be eliminated altogether. The risk of deficiencies may be low, but if you're strict about the diet, it can work wonders.

A Word on CBD

Marijuana, or cannabis, is a plant originally from Central Asia that has been used for medicinal purposes for at least 3,000 years. Because the marijuana plant contains chemicals that may help or treat a range of illnesses and symptoms, many people argue that it should be legal for medical purposes. More than half of US states have legalized marijuana in some form, but the FDA still hasn't approved of its use as a medicine.

There are two main cannabinoids found in the marijuana plant: THC (tetrahydrocannabinol) and CBD (cannabidiol). CBD and THC have the exact same molecular structure, but a slight difference in how the atoms are arranged accounts for the differing impacts on your body. Both CBD and THC are chemically similar to your body's own endocannabinoids, which allows them to interact with your cannabinoid receptors. The interaction impacts the release of neurotransmitters in your brain. Neurotransmitters are chemicals responsible for relaying messages between cells. The main difference between CBD and THC is that CBD does not induce a high whereas THC does.

CBD has been proven to help with illnesses like epilepsy, fibromyalgia, and even certain cancers. New studies also show that CBD can help or even treat chronic diseases such as diabetes, depression, multiple sclerosis, inflammation, and chronic pain.

I used cannabis to treat my chronic nerve pain, and I believe that it helped me with my nerve damage and inflammation. Research shows that there is very low toxicity in and little to no possibility of addiction to medical marijuana taken in low therapeutic doses. I advise readers to learn more before ingesting it.

POSTSCRIPT FROM DR. FAWAZ

All autoimmune diseases are caused by a betrayal of the immune system. The immune system starts targeting normal body cells with the same lethal force as it would target a virus, bacteria, or parasite. This happens because of autoantibodies.

Autoimmune disease is the result of the interaction between the genes and the environment. Many different genes increase vulnerability or susceptibility to autoimmune disease. Unfortunately, only a small number of those genes have been identified.

Environmental triggers include, but are not limited to, all of the following: stress; exposure to chemicals; pollutants; toxins; bacterial, viral, and fungal parasites; hormones; diet; micronutrient deficiencies; drugs; weight gain; and UVB radiation exposure.

Some of those factors can be easy to control such as diet, stress, and sleep. Others are more challenging or impossible to control such as genetics and infection history.

One of the common threads among all autoimmune diseases is a leaky gut, or as it is known in the scientific literature, gut permeability. The gut lining is made of a single-cell layer that acts as a barrier that does not allow food to cross into the bloodstream until it has been digested and broken down to its simplest components. Those cells are held together by a protein that forms a strong bond between them, forming tight junctions. Due to any of the environmental triggers mentioned earlier, damage can occur in the tight junction or in the cells themselves, creating holes that allow partially digested food or viruses and bacteria to cross from inside the gut to the bloodstream. The body then starts attacking the partially digested food and creates antibodies against those foods.

The problem is a phenomenon called "molecular mimicry." When the body starts forming antibodies against partially digested foods or viruses and bacteria, those antibodies start to attack the body itself. For example, when the body creates antibodies against gluten, those antibodies start attacking the thyroid. Leaky gut is the common thread in all autoimmune diseases, and gluten causes leaky gut in everyone, whether or not you have celiac disease.

When it comes to dealing with autoimmune diseases, dealing with the root cause of the problem is crucial. It starts with proper testing because everybody is different. I personally prefer food sensitivity and allergy testing so I can learn exactly what foods are causing inflammation in your body.

In addition to food, we need to find out what is going on with the gut microbiome. A healthy gut microbiome is crucial for our health. Gut bacteria are important for digesting food, breaking down micronutrients, absorbing nutrients, dealing with pathogenic bacterial or yeast, and more. A comprehensive stool analysis can give us a good picture of what is going on with the gut microbiome health.

Furthermore, we need to focus on regulating blood sugar and adrenal function. Blood sugar fluctuation can cause systemic inflammation and gut damage.

Last but not least, we need to regulate the immune system. Leaky gut, hormone imbalances, nutrient deficiency, and inflammation all contribute to immune system dysfunction. By repairing the gut, removing food-borne immune triggers, eating nutrient-dense foods, and supporting blood sugar, the autoimmune diet helps support healthy immune function.

ACKNOWLEDGMENTS

I'd like to thank all the people in my life who have helped me battle my way back to health. Dr. Fawaz obviously deserves the bulk of the praise, at least when it comes to helping me know what decisions to make and why. Dr. Fawaz isn't just a brilliant healer; he's also a compassionate human being who genuinely wants his patients to get well. He routinely worked with me on his breaks, and there were times when I was at his office learning from him for hours. Thank you, Dr. Fawaz!

As far as emotional support goes, no one can top my husband, Arjun. He is my rock, and without him, you wouldn't be reading these words. His insistence that we get out of the house that fateful day led to my accidental discovery of Dr. Fawaz at that mall, and that chance encounter changed my life. Besides that one lucky day, Arjun has also been there for me at every step of the way. I could write a whole book about how much I love him, but I'm not sure anyone would want to read it but me!

My parents have also been a source of love and support throughout my journey to health, which has lasted for most of my life. I'm sure it was very difficult for them to see their daughter go through major medical issues, but their strength helped me find my strength, which gave me the will to keep pushing on as I hit one roadblock after another. I love you both so very much, and I promise to come to India for visits as often as possible!

Arjun's parents and his sister-in-law have also been tremendously supportive over the past couple years. In addition to opening their home to me, they have also opened their hearts to me. His parents have always treated me like a daughter; they have never treated me with pity. I'll never forget the days when Arjun's mother held my hand when I couldn't walk. Thank you so much for making me feel like part of the family!

Thank you also to my editor, Jeremy Elvis Herman, who chiseled the rough edges off my words and polished my sentences.

Last but not the least, I'd like to thank Shravanji, who has been a father figure to me. He pointed me toward the right path, and I know I'll always have his blessings.

And thank you to all the other beautiful people in my life who have helped me stay strong. I love you all!

MORE ABOUT BAINTI

For more information about Bainti Parmar's amazing transformation, for yummy plant-based recipes, and for general information about food and cannabis, please visit www.thesillycilantro.com. Please also feel free to contact Bainti at info@thesillycilantro.com.

PLEASE CONSULT YOUR DOCTOR

Before you make any major changes in your lifestyle, please consult your doctor.

Made in United States
Orlando, FL
04 November 2026

90203406R00046